Guide to Total Body Transformation

How to Lose weight, Build Muscle, and Improve Endurance in Just 12 Weeks for a Fitter and Healthier You

---

Maya Harmony

CONTENTS

The Philosophy of Total Body Transformation

Welcome to **"Guide to Total Body Transformation."** My name is Maya Harmony and I designed this book to be your comprehensive guide on a journey toward a healthier, fitter, and more vibrant you. The philosophy of total body transformation is not just about losing weight or building muscle; it's about embracing a holistic approach to health and wellness that encompasses the mind, body, and spirit.

At its core, total body transformation is rooted in the belief that true change comes from within. It's about setting realistic and achievable goals, understanding the science behind physical changes, and fostering a positive mindset that supports your journey. This philosophy recognizes that each person's path to fitness is unique, and it encourages you to listen to your body, adjust as needed, and celebrate every milestone along the way.

Throughout this book, you will learn how to create a personalized plan that suits your specific needs and goals. You'll gain insights into the fundamentals of nutrition and exercise, understand how to track and adjust your progress, and discover strategies to maintain your transformation long after the 12 weeks are over.

This journey will challenge you, but it will also empower you. By the end of this book, you will not only have transformed your body but also cultivated a healthier lifestyle and mindset that can sustain you for years to come. So, let's embark on this exciting adventure together and unlock the fitter, healthier you that's waiting within.

Setting Realistic and Achievable Goals

Embarking on a journey of total body transformation requires setting realistic and achievable goals. These goals serve as the foundation of your success, guiding your efforts and keeping you motivated throughout the 12-week program.

Realistic goals are those that are attainable within the given timeframe, considering your starting point, lifestyle, and individual capabilities. They are specific, measurable, and broken down into manageable steps. For example, instead of aiming to lose 30 pounds in a month, a more realistic goal might be to lose 1-2 pounds per week. This approach not only sets you up for success but also promotes healthy, sustainable weight loss.

Achievable goals are ones that you believe you can accomplish with consistent effort and dedication. They take into account your current fitness level, resources, and potential obstacles. Setting achievable goals helps prevent discouragement and burnout, allowing you to maintain a positive mindset and stay committed to your journey.

By setting realistic and achievable goals, you create a clear roadmap for your transformation. These goals provide direction, focus, and a sense of purpose, making the process more manageable and enjoyable. Remember, each small victory brings you closer to your ultimate goal of a fitter and healthier you.

Understanding the Science Behind Weight Loss, Muscle Gain, and Endurance

Achieving a total body transformation involves more than just working out and eating well; it requires a deep understanding of the underlying science. By grasping the principles behind weight loss, muscle gain, and endurance, you can optimize your efforts and make informed decisions that lead to sustainable results.

Weight Loss

Weight loss fundamentally revolves around the concept of energy balance, which is the relationship between the calories you consume and the calories you expend. To lose weight, you need to create a calorie deficit, meaning you burn more calories than you consume. This can be achieved through a combination of diet and exercise:

- **Diet:** Reducing caloric intake by consuming nutrient-dense foods that are lower in calories but high in vitamins, minerals, and other essential nutrients. This approach ensures you get the necessary nutrients without excessive calories.

- **Exercise:** Increasing caloric expenditure through physical activity. Both aerobic exercises (like running, cycling, and swimming) and anaerobic exercises (like weight lifting and high-intensity interval training) are effective for burning calories.

It's important to note that extreme caloric deficits can lead to muscle loss and a slower metabolism. Therefore, aiming for a moderate calorie deficit is more sustainable and healthier in the long term.

Muscle Gain

Muscle gain, or hypertrophy, occurs when your muscles repair and grow stronger after being subjected to resistance training. This process involves several key factors:

- **Progressive Overload:** Continuously challenging your muscles by increasing the weight, reps, or intensity of your workouts. This stimulates muscle fibers to adapt and grow.

- **Protein Intake:** Consuming adequate protein is

essential for muscle repair and growth. Protein provides the building blocks (amino acids) needed for muscle synthesis. Aim for a protein-rich diet that includes sources like lean meats, dairy, legumes, and plant-based proteins.

- **Rest and Recovery:** Muscles grow during rest periods, not while you are working out. Ensuring you get enough sleep and allowing time for muscle groups to recover between workouts is crucial for muscle growth.

Balancing these factors helps promote muscle hypertrophy while minimizing the risk of injury and overtraining.

Endurance

Endurance refers to the ability to sustain physical activity over extended periods. Improving endurance involves enhancing both cardiovascular and muscular endurance:

- **Cardiovascular Endurance:** This is the ability of your heart, lungs, and circulatory system to supply oxygen to your muscles during prolonged exercise. It can be improved through consistent aerobic exercise, such as running, cycling, or swimming. Training at various intensities, including steady-state and interval training, helps enhance cardiovascular efficiency.

- **Muscular Endurance:** This is the ability of your muscles to perform repetitive contractions over time without fatigue. It can be improved through resistance training with lighter weights and higher repetitions, as well as activities like circuit training and bodyweight exercises.

Understanding the interplay between these elements allows you to design a comprehensive fitness program that addresses all aspects of your transformation. By applying the principles of energy balance, progressive overload, and endurance training, you can effectively lose weight, build muscle, and improve your overall fitness.

Comprehending the science behind weight loss, muscle

gain, and endurance equips you with the knowledge to make strategic choices in your fitness journey. This understanding fosters a more efficient and effective approach, ensuring that your efforts lead to a successful and sustainable transformation.

Chapter 1: Preparing for Your Transformation

Assessing Your Starting Point

Before embarking on any fitness journey, it's crucial to understand your starting point. Assessing your current fitness level, body composition, and overall health provides a baseline from which you can measure progress. This initial assessment not only helps in setting realistic and achievable goals but also tailors your workout and nutrition plan to suit your unique needs. By knowing where you stand, you can chart a clear path forward and stay motivated as you witness your transformation unfold.

Baseline Fitness Assessment

The baseline fitness assessment is a comprehensive evaluation of your current physical condition. It includes several key components:

1. Cardiovascular Fitness

2. Muscular Strength and Endurance

3. Flexibility

4. Body Composition

Each of these areas provides valuable insights into your overall fitness and helps identify strengths and areas for improvement.

1. Cardiovascular Fitness

Cardiovascular fitness refers to how well your heart, lungs, and circulatory system work together to supply oxygen during sustained physical activity. A common way to assess this is through a simple test like the 3-minute step test or a 1-mile walk/run:

- **3-Minute Step Test:** Step up and down on a platform for three minutes at a steady pace. Immediately after, measure your heart rate. The quicker your heart rate returns to normal, the better your cardiovascular fitness.

- **Mile Walk/Run:** Measure the time it takes to walk or run a mile. Record your time and heart rate at the end. This test gauges your aerobic capacity and endurance.

2. Muscular Strength and Endurance

Muscular strength is the maximum amount of force a muscle can produce, while muscular endurance is the ability of a muscle to sustain repeated contractions over time. You can assess these through various exercises:

- ❖ **Strength Test:** Perform exercises like push-ups and squats to measure how many repetitions you can do until muscle fatigue. This test helps identify your upper and lower body strength.

- ❖ **Endurance Test:** Exercises such as plank holds or sit-ups for a specified time period can assess how long your muscles can sustain effort.

3. Flexibility

Flexibility is the range of motion available at your joints. It's crucial for overall mobility and injury prevention. Common tests include:

- ❖ **Sit-and-Reach Test:** Sit on the floor with your legs straight. Reach forward as far as possible and measure the distance between your fingertips and your toes. This test primarily assesses the flexibility of your lower back and hamstrings.

Body Composition

Body composition measures the proportion of fat and non-fat mass in your body. Several methods can be used to assess this:

* **Body Mass Index (BMI):** A simple calculation using your height and weight. Although it doesn't differentiate between muscle and fat, it gives a general idea of your body weight status.

* **Body Measurements:** Use a tape measure to record the circumference of different body parts (e.g., waist, hips, arms). Tracking these measurements over time helps monitor changes in body composition.

* **Body Fat Percentage:** More accurate methods like skinfold calipers, bioelectrical impedance scales, or DEXA scans provide a detailed analysis of body fat versus lean mass.

Recording and Interpreting Results

Once you've completed your baseline fitness assessment, record your results in a dedicated journal or digital tracker. This data serves as a reference point, allowing you to track your progress throughout the 12-week program.

Interpreting these results helps you understand your starting point and identify specific areas to focus on. For instance, if your cardiovascular fitness is lower than desired, you might prioritize aerobic exercises in your routine. If you find that your flexibility is limited, incorporating regular stretching and mobility exercises can be beneficial.

By thoroughly assessing your starting point, you set the stage for a personalized and effective transformation plan. This foundational step ensures that your efforts are aligned with your current capabilities and goals, paving the way for a successful journey toward a fitter, healthier you.

Setting SMART Goals

Setting SMART goals is a powerful method to ensure your fitness journey is focused, measurable, and attainable. SMART is an acronym that stands for Specific, Measurable, Achievable, Relevant, and Time-bound.

- ❖ **Specific:** Your goals should be clear and precise. Instead of saying, **"I want to get fit,"** define what that means for you. For example, **"I want to lose 10 pounds,"** or **"I want to run a 5K."**

- ❖ **Measurable:** Ensure your goals can be tracked and measured. This helps you monitor progress and stay motivated. For instance, "I want to lose 10 pounds" is measurable, as you can track weight loss over time.

- ❖ **Achievable:** Set realistic goals that are attainable given your current fitness level and lifestyle. Aim for progress that challenges you but is still within reach, such as **"I will increase my bench press by 10 pounds in the next month."**

- ❖ **Relevant:** Your goals should align with your

overall objectives and be meaningful to you. Ensure they reflect what you truly want to achieve, like improving your health or increasing your strength.

❖ **Time-bound:** Set a specific timeframe for achieving your goals. This creates a sense of urgency and helps maintain focus. For example, **"I will lose 10 pounds in 12 weeks"** sets a clear deadline.

By setting SMART goals, you create a structured and clear path toward your fitness transformation, enhancing your likelihood of success and making your journey more rewarding.

Creating Your Personalized Plan

Creating a personalized plan is essential for achieving a successful body transformation. A one-size-fits-all approach seldom works, as individual differences in body type, fitness level, and lifestyle influence how each person responds to diet and exercise. This section guides you through understanding your body type, tailoring your nutrition to your goals, and designing a balanced workout plan. By customizing your approach, you ensure that your efforts are effective and sustainable, paving the way for lasting change.

Understanding Your Body Type

Your body type, also known as somatotype, plays a significant role in how you respond to diet and exercise. There are three primary body types: ectomorph, mesomorph, and endomorph. Each type has unique characteristics that influence your metabolism, muscle development, and fat storage. Understanding your body type helps you tailor your fitness and nutrition plan to optimize results.

Ectomorph

Ectomorphs are typically slim with a light build, narrow shoulders, and fast metabolism. They often find it hard to gain weight and muscle.

- ❖ **Diet and Exercise Tips:** Focus on consuming more calories, particularly from protein and healthy fats, to support muscle growth. Strength training with heavier weights and lower repetitions can help build muscle mass. Limit excessive cardio to avoid burning too many calories.

Mesomorph

Mesomorphs have a naturally athletic build with a more muscular frame and balanced metabolism. They tend to gain muscle easily and maintain a lower body fat percentage.

- ❖ **Diet and Exercise Tips:** A balanced diet with moderate amounts of protein, carbs, and fats works well. Combine strength training with both heavy and moderate weights and include a mix of cardio exercises to maintain overall fitness. Adjust calorie intake based on activity level to avoid excess weight gain.

Endomorph

Endomorphs often have a rounder, softer physique and a slower metabolism. They tend to store fat more easily and may find it challenging to lose weight.

- ❖ **Diet and Exercise Tips:** Focus on a diet that is lower in carbs and higher in protein and healthy fats to help manage weight. Incorporate regular cardio exercises to boost metabolism and promote fat loss. Strength training with higher repetitions can help build lean muscle and support fat burning.

By understanding your body type, you can make informed choices about your diet and exercise routines, ensuring that your personalized plan is effective and aligns with your unique needs. This foundational knowledge empowers you to work with your body's natural tendencies rather than against them, making your fitness journey more efficient and enjoyable.

Tailoring Nutrition to Your Goals

Tailoring your nutrition to your specific fitness goals is crucial for achieving a successful body transformation. Whether your goal is to lose weight, build muscle, or improve endurance, your diet plays a key role in providing the necessary fuel and nutrients.

Weight Loss

To lose weight, focus on creating a calorie deficit by consuming fewer calories than you burn. Prioritize nutrient-dense foods that are low in calories but high in vitamins, minerals, and fiber. Incorporate plenty of vegetables, fruits, lean proteins, and whole grains into your diet. Avoid processed foods, sugary snacks, and high-calorie beverages. Consistent, small changes in your diet can lead to sustainable weight loss.

Muscle Gain

Building muscle requires a calorie surplus, meaning you need to consume more calories than you burn, with an emphasis on protein. Aim to include high-quality protein sources in every meal, such as lean meats, fish, eggs, dairy, legumes, and plant-based proteins. Carbohydrates are also important to provide energy for workouts, so include whole grains, fruits, and vegetables. Healthy fats from sources like nuts, seeds, and avocados support overall health and hormone production.

Improving Endurance

For improving endurance, focus on a balanced diet rich in carbohydrates to provide sustained energy. Include whole grains, fruits, and vegetables to ensure you have enough glycogen stores for long-duration activities. Proteins are essential for muscle repair and recovery, so include them in your diet as well. Stay hydrated and consider timing your meals and snacks around your training sessions to optimize performance and recovery.

By tailoring your nutrition to your specific goals, you provide your body with the appropriate fuel and nutrients it needs to perform optimally and achieve your desired results. Understanding the role of different macronutrients and making informed food choices will enhance your progress and help you reach your fitness objectives more efficiently.

Designing a Balanced Workout Plan

Designing a balanced workout plan is essential for achieving comprehensive fitness results. A well-rounded plan incorporates various types of exercise to address different aspects of physical health, including strength, cardiovascular fitness, and flexibility.

Strength Training

Strength training builds muscle, increases metabolism, and enhances overall strength. Include exercises that target all major muscle groups: legs, back, chest, shoulders, arms, and core. Utilize a mix of free weights, machines, and bodyweight exercises. Aim for at least two to three strength training sessions per week, progressively increasing the weight and intensity to continue challenging your muscles.

Cardiovascular Training

Cardiovascular exercises improve heart health, endurance, and calorie burning. Incorporate a variety of cardio activities such as running, cycling, swimming, or group fitness classes. Aim for at least 150 minutes of moderate-intensity cardio or 75 minutes of high-intensity cardio each week. Mixing steady-state cardio with high-intensity interval training (HIIT) can provide comprehensive cardiovascular benefits.

Flexibility and Mobility

Flexibility and mobility exercises enhance your range of motion, prevent injuries, and aid in recovery. Include activities such as stretching, yoga, or Pilates in your routine. Aim to incorporate flexibility training into your workout plan at least two to three times per week, focusing on all major muscle groups.

Rest and Recovery

Rest and recovery are vital components of a balanced workout plan. Ensure you have at least one to two rest days per week to allow your muscles to repair and grow. Listen to your body and include active recovery activities, such as light stretching or walking, to promote circulation and reduce soreness.

By designing a balanced workout plan that includes strength training, cardiovascular exercise, flexibility, and adequate rest, you create a comprehensive approach to fitness. This balance ensures that you improve in all areas of physical health, leading to a more effective and sustainable body transformation.

Mindset and Motivation

Mindset and motivation are crucial elements of a successful body transformation journey. Developing a positive mindset and staying motivated can make a significant difference in achieving your fitness goals. A positive mindset involves cultivating healthy attitudes, beliefs, and habits that support your journey. Motivation, on the other hand, fuels your commitment and perseverance through challenges and setbacks.

Developing a Positive Mindset

A positive mindset is the foundation for sustainable change and growth in your fitness journey. It involves adopting constructive thoughts and attitudes that empower you to overcome obstacles and stay focused on your goals.

Key Strategies:

1. Set Realistic Expectations: Understand that progress takes time and setbacks are normal. Celebrate small victories along the way.

2. Practice Self-Compassion: Be kind to yourself and

avoid self-criticism. Acknowledge your efforts and successes, no matter how small.

3. Focus on the Process: Emphasize the journey rather than just the end goal. Enjoy the daily improvements and learning experiences.

4. Visualize Success: Create a mental image of achieving your goals. Visualizing success can boost confidence and motivation.

5. Surround Yourself with Support: Build a support network of friends, family, or fitness buddies who encourage and inspire you.

6. Stay Flexible: Adapt to changes and setbacks with resilience. Learn from challenges and adjust your approach as needed.

By cultivating a positive mindset, you enhance your ability to stay committed and resilient throughout your body transformation journey. This mental strength not only supports your physical efforts but also fosters a healthier relationship with fitness and self-improvement.

Overcoming Common Barriers

Embarking on a body transformation journey often comes with challenges that can hinder progress. Recognizing and overcoming these common barriers is essential for maintaining momentum and achieving your fitness goals.

Lack of Time

Strategy: Prioritize and schedule your workouts like appointments. Opt for shorter, high-intensity workouts if time is limited. Incorporate physical activity into your daily routine, such as taking the stairs instead of the elevator or walking during lunch breaks.

Lack of Motivation

Strategy: Set clear and meaningful goals to keep yourself motivated. Find activities you enjoy and vary your routine to prevent boredom. Seek inspiration from others, join fitness communities, or work with a personal trainer for accountability and support.

Poor Nutrition Choices

Strategy: Plan and prepare meals ahead of time to avoid relying on unhealthy options. Keep nutritious snacks readily available. Educate yourself about balanced nutrition and make informed food choices that align with your goals.

Fatigue or Burnout

Strategy: Ensure adequate rest and recovery between workouts. Listen to your body and adjust your intensity or frequency of exercise as needed. Incorporate relaxation techniques, such as yoga or meditation, to reduce stress and rejuvenate your mind and body.

Lack of Support

Strategy: Surround yourself with supportive individuals who encourage and motivate you. Share your goals with friends and family who can provide emotional support. Consider joining online forums or local fitness groups to connect with like-minded individuals.

Plateaus

Strategy: Plateaus are normal in any fitness journey. Evaluate your routine and consider adjusting your workouts or nutrition plan. Set new challenges or goals to keep yourself engaged and motivated. Track your progress to recognize improvements beyond the scale.

By proactively addressing these common barriers, you can maintain consistency and focus on your body transformation goals. Remember, persistence and determination are key to overcoming obstacles and achieving long-term success in your fitness journey.

Chapter 2: Nutrition for Transformation

Nutrition is a cornerstone of achieving a successful body transformation. It fuels your workouts, supports muscle growth, and enhances overall health. This section focuses on understanding the fundamentals of nutrition, including macronutrients (proteins, carbohydrates, and fats), micronutrients (vitamins and minerals), and the importance of hydration. By mastering these fundamentals, you can optimize your diet to support your fitness goals and maintain long-term health.

Fundamentals of Nutrition

Macronutrients: Proteins, Carbs, and Fats

Proteins:

Role: Proteins are essential for building and repairing tissues, including muscles, bones, skin, and organs.

- ❖ **Sources:** Include lean meats (chicken, turkey, lean cuts of beef), fish, eggs, dairy products (Greek yogurt, cottage cheese), legumes (beans, lentils), and plant-based proteins (tofu, tempeh, quinoa).

❖ **Recommended Intake:** Aim to include a source of protein in each meal to support muscle recovery and growth.

Carbohydrates:

Role: Carbohydrates are the body's primary source of energy, especially during exercise.

❖ **Sources:** Opt for complex carbohydrates such as whole grains (brown rice, oats, whole wheat), fruits, vegetables, and legumes. These provide sustained energy and fiber.

❖ **Recommended Intake:** Prioritize whole, unprocessed carbohydrates over refined sugars and flours. Adjust intake based on activity level and energy needs.

Fats:

Role: Healthy fats are vital for hormone production, brain function, and absorption of fat-soluble vitamins (A, D, E, K).

❖ **Sources:** Include unsaturated fats from sources like nuts, seeds, avocados, olive oil, and fatty fish (salmon, mackerel).

* **Recommended Intake:** Balance intake of saturated fats (found in animal products) with unsaturated fats to support heart health and overall well-being.

Micronutrients: Vitamins and Minerals

* **Vitamins:**

Role: Vitamins play crucial roles in various bodily functions, including immune function, energy production, and tissue repair.

* **Sources:** Obtain vitamins from a balanced diet that includes a variety of fruits, vegetables, whole grains, and lean proteins.

* **Key Vitamins:** Vitamin C (found in citrus fruits, bell peppers), Vitamin D (sunlight exposure, fortified dairy products), Vitamin B complex (whole grains, leafy greens).

Minerals:

Role: Minerals are essential for bone health, nerve

function, muscle contraction, and fluid balance.

- ❖ **Sources:** Include minerals like calcium (dairy products, leafy greens), iron (red meat, beans, fortified cereals), potassium (bananas, potatoes), and magnesium (nuts, seeds, whole grains).

- ❖ **Key Minerals:** Ensure adequate intake through a varied diet to support overall health and prevent deficiencies.

Hydration and Its Importance

Role:

- ❖ **Importance:** Hydration is critical for regulating body temperature, lubricating joints, delivering nutrients to cells, and removing waste products.

- ❖ **Sources:** Water is the best source of hydration, but fluids from fruits, vegetables, and beverages like herbal teas also contribute.

- ❖ **Daily Intake:** Aim to drink at least 8 glasses (about 2 liters) of water per day, adjusting for physical activity and climate.

Understanding the fundamentals of nutrition, including macronutrients, micronutrients, and hydration, empowers you to make informed food choices that support your body transformation goals. By prioritizing a balanced diet rich in whole foods and adequate hydration, you provide your body with the nutrients it needs to thrive, perform optimally during workouts, and achieve lasting results in your fitness journey.

Meal Planning and Prep

A weekly meal plan helps you stay organized, save time, and make healthier food choices.

Steps:

1. Set Goals: Define your nutritional goals (e.g., weight loss, muscle gain, maintenance).

2. Plan Meals: Designate specific meals for each day (breakfast, lunch, dinner, snacks).

3. Include Variety: Incorporate a balance of macronutrients (proteins, carbs, fats) and micronutrients (vitamins, minerals).

4. Consider Preferences: Choose recipes and foods you

enjoy to maintain satisfaction and adherence.

5. Prep Ahead: Plan for leftovers or batch cooking to streamline meal preparation.

Grocery Shopping Tips

Plan your shopping list based on your meal plan to avoid impulse purchases.

Healthy Choices:

Focus on fresh produce, lean proteins, whole grains, and healthy fats.

Budgeting:

Compare prices, use coupons, and consider buying in bulk for cost-effective options.

Read Labels:

Check nutritional labels to make informed choices about packaged foods.

Time-Saving Meal Prep Strategies

Batch Cooking:

Prepare large quantities of staple foods (e.g., grains,

proteins) to use throughout the week.

Pre-cut and Wash:

Wash and chop vegetables in advance for quick meal assembly.

Portion Control:

Divide meals into individual portions for easy grab-and-go options.

Use Convenience Items:

Utilize pre-cut veggies, canned beans, or frozen fruits for efficiency without sacrificing nutrition.

Meal planning and preparation are essential tools for maintaining a nutritious diet that supports your body transformation goals. By creating a weekly meal plan, practicing efficient grocery shopping, and implementing time-saving meal prep strategies, you can establish healthy eating habits that are sustainable and enjoyable. These practices not only save time but also ensure that you have nutritious meals readily available, making it easier to stay on track with your fitness journey and achieve long-term success.

Special Diets and Adjustments

Special diets cater to specific dietary preferences, restrictions, or health conditions, ensuring individuals can meet their nutritional needs while achieving their fitness goals. Understanding various dietary options allows you to make informed choices that align with your lifestyle and optimize your body transformation journey.

Vegetarian and Vegan Options

Vegetarian

A vegetarian diet excludes meat, poultry, and seafood but may include dairy products and eggs.

Key Considerations:

- **Protein Sources:** Incorporate plant-based proteins such as beans, lentils, tofu, tempeh, nuts, and seeds.

- **Iron and B12:** Ensure adequate intake through sources

like leafy greens, fortified cereals, and dairy products (for lacto-vegetarians).

- **Omega-3 Fatty Acids:** Include sources like flaxseeds, chia seeds, and walnuts for essential fats.

Vegan

A vegan diet excludes all animal products, including meat, dairy, eggs, and often honey.

Key Considerations:

- **Protein Sources:** Rely on plant-based proteins such as legumes, tofu, tempeh, quinoa, and plant-based protein powders.

- **Vitamin B12:** Supplement or consume fortified foods like nutritional yeast or fortified plant milks.

- **Calcium and Vitamin D:** Include fortified plant milks and cereals, leafy greens (e.g., kale, collard greens), and exposure to sunlight for vitamin D synthesis.

Choosing a vegetarian or vegan diet requires careful planning to ensure you meet your nutritional needs while supporting your body transformation goals. By incorporating a variety of plant-based foods rich in essential nutrients, you can maintain optimal health, energy levels, and performance throughout your fitness journey. Adjustments based on individual preferences and dietary restrictions can empower you to achieve sustainable results while adhering to your chosen lifestyle.

Low-Carb and Keto Diets

Low-Carb Diet:

A low-carb diet restricts carbohydrates, emphasizing proteins and fats.

- **Purpose:** Promotes weight loss by reducing insulin levels and increasing fat burning.

- **Foods to Eat:** Lean meats, fish, eggs, non-starchy vegetables, nuts, seeds.

- **Foods to Limit:** Sugary foods, grains, fruits, starchy vegetables.

- **Benefits:** Effective for weight loss, improved blood sugar control, and increased satiety.

Keto Diet (Ketogenic Diet):

A very low-carb, high-fat diet that induces ketosis, where the body burns fat for fuel.

- **Purpose:** Rapid weight loss, improved mental clarity, and enhanced energy levels.

- **Foods to Eat:** High-fat foods like avocados, butter, olive oil, fatty meats, and low-carb vegetables.

- **Foods to Avoid:** High-carb foods such as grains, sugars, fruits, and most legumes.

- **Benefits:** Effective for weight loss, managing epilepsy, and controlling blood sugar levels in diabetes.

Considerations:

- **Nutrient Balance:** Ensure adequate intake of vitamins, minerals, and fiber.

- **Long-Term Sustainability:** Plan meals carefully to meet nutritional needs without compromising health.

- **Consultation:** Consult with a healthcare professional before starting to ensure suitability and safety.

Both diets can be effective for weight loss and certain health conditions but require careful planning to ensure nutritional adequacy and long-term sustainability.

Managing Food Allergies and Intolerances

Managing food allergies and intolerances is crucial for maintaining health and well-being, especially during a body transformation journey. Here are key considerations:

* **Identify Trigger Foods:** Determine specific foods that trigger allergic reactions or intolerances through elimination diets or allergy testing.

* **Read Labels:** Always read food labels carefully to avoid allergens or ingredients that may cause reactions.

* **Alternative Options:** Substitute allergenic foods with safe alternatives that provide similar nutritional benefits.

* **Consult a Registered Dietitian:** Seek guidance

from a healthcare professional, such as a registered dietitian, to create a balanced diet plan that meets your nutritional needs while avoiding allergens.

❖ **Communicate Clearly:** When dining out or attending events, communicate your food allergies or intolerances to ensure safe food preparation.

By managing food allergies and intolerances effectively, you can maintain a healthy diet that supports your body transformation goals while preventing adverse reactions.

Supplements: Do You Need Them?

Supplements are products designed to complement your diet by providing additional nutrients that may be lacking or needed in higher amounts for specific health or fitness goals. While they can be beneficial, especially in certain situations, they are not a substitute for a balanced diet rich in whole foods.

Protein Supplements

Protein supplements are convenient sources of protein, particularly useful for individuals who struggle to meet their protein needs through diet alone.

Types:

- **Whey Protein:** Derived from milk, whey protein is quickly absorbed and ideal for post-workout recovery.

- **Plant-Based Protein:** Made from sources like peas, rice, or hemp, suitable for vegetarians and vegans.

- **Casein Protein:** Absorbed more slowly, providing sustained amino acid release.

Usage:

Use protein supplements to enhance muscle recovery

and growth, especially after workouts when protein synthesis is heightened.

Vitamins and Minerals

Vitamins and minerals supplements are used to fill gaps in nutrient intake or to support specific health needs.

Types:

- **Multivitamins:** Provide a broad spectrum of essential vitamins and minerals.

- **Single Nutrient Supplements:** Target specific deficiencies, such as Vitamin D or Iron supplements.

Usage:

Consider supplements when dietary intake is inadequate or when specific health conditions require higher nutrient levels.

Performance Enhancers

Performance enhancers are supplements designed to improve athletic performance, endurance, or recovery.

Types:

- **Creatine:** Helps increase muscle mass, strength, and

exercise performance.

- **Caffeine:** Enhances focus, endurance, and fat metabolism during exercise.

- **Beta-Alanine:** Delays muscle fatigue and improves high-intensity exercise capacity.

Usage:

Use performance enhancers under guidance and according to recommended dosages to maximize benefits and minimize risks.

While supplements can support your fitness goals, they should complement a well-balanced diet and not replace it. Consider supplements based on your individual needs, goals, and dietary habits. Consult with a healthcare professional or registered dietitian to determine if supplements are appropriate for you and to ensure safe and effective usage.

Chapter 3: Exercise for Transformation

Exercise is a cornerstone of achieving a successful body transformation. Part III focuses on the essentials of exercise, including different types of exercise, understanding key terms like reps and sets, and the importance of warm-up and cool-down routines. By mastering these fundamentals, you can design an effective workout regimen that supports your fitness goals and promotes overall health.

The Essentials of Exercise

Types of Exercise: Cardio, Strength, and Flexibility

Cardiovascular Exercise:

- **Purpose:** Cardio exercises, such as running, cycling, or swimming, elevate your heart rate and improve cardiovascular health.

- **Benefits:** Enhances endurance, burns calories, and supports weight management.

Strength Training:

- **Purpose:** Strength training involves lifting weights or using resistance to build muscle strength and endurance.

- Benefits: Increases muscle mass, boosts metabolism, and enhances overall strength and functional movement.

Flexibility Training:

- Purpose: Flexibility exercises like stretching or yoga improve joint range of motion and reduce the risk of injury.

- Benefits: Enhances flexibility, promotes relaxation, and supports muscle recovery.

Understanding Reps, Sets, and Rest

Repetitions (Reps):

Reps refer to the number of times you perform a specific exercise in one set.

- Purpose: Determines the muscular endurance or strength adaptation.

Sets:

Sets are groups of consecutive repetitions performed with brief rest intervals in between.

- **Purpose:** Sets allow you to achieve a specific volume of work to stimulate muscle growth or endurance.

Rest Intervals:

- **Importance:** Rest periods between sets allow muscles to recover and replenish energy stores.

- **Optimal Rest:** Adjust rest intervals based on exercise intensity and training goals (e.g., shorter rests for endurance, longer rests for strength).

Importance of Warm-Up and Cool-Down

Warm-Up:

- **Purpose:** Prepares your body for exercise by increasing heart rate, circulation, and muscle temperature.

- **Components:** Include dynamic movements, light cardio, and joint mobility exercises.

Cool-Down:

- **Purpose:** Facilitates recovery by gradually lowering heart rate and stretching muscles to prevent stiffness and injury.

- **Components:** Focus on static stretching, deep breathing, and relaxation techniques.

Understanding the essentials of exercise, including different types of exercises (cardio, strength, flexibility), key terms like reps and sets, and the importance of warm-up and cool-down routines, empowers you to design a well-rounded workout program. By incorporating variety, proper technique, and adequate recovery into your exercise routine, you can maximize results, reduce injury risk, and maintain long-term fitness progress toward your transformation goals.

Strength Training

Strength training is a fundamental component of any comprehensive fitness regimen, focusing on building muscle strength, endurance, and overall functional fitness. This section covers basic exercises, advanced techniques, and how to create a progressive strength training plan to maximize your results effectively and safely.

Basic Strength Training Exercises

Purpose:

- Basic strength training exercises target major muscle groups and lay the foundation for muscle development and overall strength.

Examples:

- Upper Body: Push-ups, dumbbell bench press, bicep curls.

- Lower Body: Squats, lunges, deadlifts.

- Core: Planks, Russian twists, leg raises.

Technique:

- Focus on proper form and controlled movements to engage targeted muscles effectively.

- Start with lighter weights or bodyweight to master technique before progressing.

Advanced Strength Training Techniques

Purpose:

- Advanced techniques challenge muscles further, promoting strength gains and muscle hypertrophy (growth).

Examples:

- **Supersets:** Alternating between two different exercises without rest.

- **Drop Sets:** Gradually reducing weight after reaching muscle fatigue.

- **Pyramid Sets:** Increasing or decreasing weight and reps in successive sets.

Technique:

- Requires familiarity with basic exercises and careful progression to avoid injury.

- Adjust intensity and volume based on fitness level and goals.

Creating a Progressive Strength Training Plan

Purpose:

- A progressive plan systematically increases workload to continually challenge muscles and promote growth.

Steps:

1. **Set Goals:** Define specific strength goals (e.g., increasing bench press weight, improving squat form).

2. **Choose Exercises:** Select exercises that target all major muscle groups for balanced development.

3. **Progression:** Gradually increase weight, reps, or intensity as strength improves.

4. **Rest and Recovery:** Allow adequate rest between sessions and incorporate recovery techniques (e.g., foam rolling, stretching).

Strength training is essential for building muscle, improving metabolism, and enhancing overall physical performance. By incorporating basic exercises, exploring advanced techniques cautiously, and following a progressive strength training plan, you can achieve significant gains in strength and muscle mass while minimizing the risk of injury. Consistency and proper technique are key to success in strength training, supporting your body transformation goals effectively over time.

Cardiovascular Training

Cardiovascular training, often referred to as cardio, plays a crucial role in improving heart health, endurance, and overall fitness levels. This section explores different types of cardio workouts, the benefits of High-Intensity Interval Training (HIIT), and methods for building endurance through steady-state cardio.

Types of Cardio Workouts

Purpose:

- Cardio exercises elevate heart rate and improve cardiovascular fitness by engaging large muscle groups.

Examples:

- **Running/Jogging:** Effective for outdoor or treadmill workouts.

- **Cycling:** Stationary bikes or outdoor cycling for lower body conditioning.

- **Swimming:** Full-body workout with low impact on joints.

- **Rowing:** Engages upper and lower body muscles simultaneously.

Technique:

- Maintain a consistent pace that challenges your cardiovascular system without overexertion.

- Choose activities you enjoy to enhance adherence and consistency.

High-Intensity Interval Training (HIIT)

Purpose:

- HIIT alternates between short bursts of intense exercise and periods of rest or lower-intensity activity.

Benefits:

- Increases calorie burn and metabolic rate both during and after exercise.

- Improves cardiovascular endurance and muscle strength in less time compared to traditional cardio.

Technique:

- **Example:** Sprinting for 30 seconds followed by 1 minute of walking or jogging.

- Adjust intensity and duration based on fitness level

and goals.

Building Endurance through Steady-State Cardio

Purpose:

- Steady-state cardio involves maintaining a moderate intensity for an extended period, improving aerobic capacity and endurance.

Examples:

- Brisk walking, jogging, cycling, or swimming at a steady pace for 20-60 minutes.

- Aim for a consistent effort level that allows sustained activity without excessive fatigue.

Technique:

- Focus on maintaining a steady pace that challenges your cardiovascular system without becoming overly fatigued.

- Gradually increase duration or intensity over time to improve endurance.

Incorporating a variety of cardio workouts, including

HIIT for intensity and steady-state cardio for endurance, enhances cardiovascular health and overall fitness. Choose activities that suit your preferences and fitness goals to ensure consistency and enjoyment in your workout routine.

By balancing different types of cardio and adjusting intensity based on your fitness level, you can achieve significant improvements in heart health, endurance, and overall well-being during your body transformation journey.

Flexibility and Mobility

Flexibility and mobility are essential components of overall fitness and well-being, contributing to improved posture, reduced risk of injury, and enhanced athletic performance. This section explores the importance of stretching, the benefits of yoga and Pilates for flexibility, and the role of daily mobility routines in maintaining optimal movement patterns.

Importance of Stretching

Purpose:

- Stretching improves muscle elasticity and joint range of motion, enhancing overall flexibility and reducing muscle tension.

Types:

- Static Stretching: Holding a stretch position for 15-30 seconds to lengthen muscles gradually.

- Dynamic Stretching: Incorporating controlled movements to prepare muscles for activity.

Benefits:

- Enhances muscle coordination and efficiency during exercise.

- Promotes relaxation and reduces the risk of muscle strains or injuries.

Yoga and Pilates for Flexibility

Purpose:

- Yoga and Pilates focus on body awareness, flexibility, and core strength through controlled movements and poses.

Yoga:

- Types: Includes various styles such as Hatha, Vinyasa, and Bikram yoga.

- Benefits: Improves flexibility, balance, and mental relaxation through breathing techniques and mindfulness.

Pilates:

- Focus: Centers on core strength, stability, and flexibility through controlled movements.

- Benefits: Enhances posture, muscle tone, and joint mobility with an emphasis on alignment and body awareness.

Daily Mobility Routines

Purpose:

- Daily mobility routines prevent stiffness, improve joint function, and maintain overall movement quality.

Components:

- **Joint Circles:** Perform gentle rotations of major joints (e.g., shoulders, hips) to lubricate and maintain mobility.

- **Foam Rolling:** Use a foam roller to release tight muscles and fascia, enhancing flexibility and reducing muscle soreness.

Benefits:

- Supports recovery and readiness for physical activity.

- Counteracts the effects of sedentary lifestyles and promotes longevity in movement capabilities.

Incorporating stretching exercises, yoga or Pilates sessions, and daily mobility routines into your fitness regimen enhances flexibility, mobility, and overall physical well-being. These practices not only improve movement quality and reduce injury risk but also contribute to relaxation and stress relief. By prioritizing flexibility and mobility exercises, you can maintain optimal function and support your body transformation goals effectively over time.

Chapter 4: Tracking and Adjusting Your Plan

Tracking your progress is essential for staying on course with your body transformation goals. This section focuses on monitoring your progress effectively through tracking weight and body measurements, utilizing fitness apps and wearables, and maintaining a workout and nutrition journal. By establishing these practices, you can assess your achievements, identify areas for improvement, and adjust your plan to optimize results.

Monitoring Progress

Tracking Weight and Body Measurements

Purpose:

- Monitoring changes in weight and body measurements provides feedback on your body composition and overall progress.

Techniques:

- Weight: Use a reliable scale to measure changes in

body weight regularly (e.g., weekly or biweekly).

- Body Measurements: Track changes in waist circumference, hips, thighs, and other key areas using a tape measure.

Benefits:

- Helps assess fat loss, muscle gain, and overall body composition changes.

- Provides motivation and accountability throughout your transformation journey.

Using Fitness Apps and Wearables

Purpose:

- Fitness apps and wearables help track exercise performance, daily activity levels, and nutritional intake.

Features:

- Exercise Tracking: Record workouts, track calories burned, and monitor progress over time.

- Activity Monitoring: Measure daily steps, distance traveled, and active minutes to maintain consistent activity levels.

- Nutrition Logging: Log meals, track macronutrient intake, and monitor hydration to support dietary goals.

Benefits:

- Enhances motivation by visualizing progress and achievements.

- Provides insights into trends and patterns to make informed adjustments to your fitness and nutrition plan.

Keeping a Workout and Nutrition Journal

Purpose:

- A workout and nutrition journal helps you record and analyze your daily activities, workouts, and dietary choices.

Components:

- Workout Log: Document exercises, sets, reps, and weights used during strength training sessions.

- Nutrition Log: Record meals, snacks, portion sizes, and nutritional content to monitor dietary habits.

Benefits:

- Promotes accountability and consistency in following your exercise and nutrition plan.

- Identifies areas for improvement and adjustments based on recorded data and progress.

Tracking and adjusting your plan through monitoring progress, utilizing fitness apps and wearables, and maintaining a workout and nutrition journal are integral to achieving and sustaining your body transformation goals.

These practices provide valuable insights into your journey, allowing you to make informed decisions, stay motivated, and optimize your efforts towards long-term success. By implementing these monitoring strategies consistently, you can adapt your plan effectively to overcome challenges and continue progressing towards a healthier and fitter lifestyle.

Adjusting Your Plan

Adjusting your fitness and nutrition plan is crucial for overcoming challenges, achieving sustained progress, and maintaining motivation throughout your body transformation journey. This section focuses on identifying plateaus, tweaking nutrition strategies, and modifying workouts to effectively navigate obstacles and optimize results.

Identifying Plateaus and Making Adjustments

Recognition:

- Plateaus occur when progress slows or halts despite consistent effort and adherence to your plan.

Indicators:

- Lack of changes in weight, body measurements, or performance improvements.

- Decreased motivation or enthusiasm for workouts.

Strategies:

- Assess Progress: Review tracking data (weight, measurements, performance logs) to identify patterns or stagnation points.

- Adjust Caloric Intake: Modify calorie consumption to support continued fat loss or muscle gain, based on current goals and metabolic needs.

- Change Exercise Routine: Introduce new exercises, vary intensity, or adjust volume to stimulate muscle adaptation and break through plateaus.

Tweaking Nutrition for Continued Progress

Evaluation:

- Evaluate current dietary habits and nutrient intake to ensure alignment with fitness goals and metabolic demands.

Adjustments:

- Caloric Balance: Fine-tune calorie intake to maintain a slight deficit for weight loss or surplus for muscle gain.

- Macro Distribution: Adjust macronutrient ratios (protein, carbs, fats) based on performance and recovery needs.

- Meal Timing: Consider nutrient timing around workouts to optimize energy levels and recovery.

Modifying Workouts to Overcome Stagnation

Assessment:

- Review workout logs, performance metrics, and feedback to identify areas of stagnation or limited progress.

Strategies:

- Progressive Overload: Gradually increase weights, reps, or intensity to challenge muscles and stimulate growth.

- Variation: Incorporate different exercises, training modalities (e.g., HIIT, circuit training), or equipment to keep workouts engaging and effective.

- Recovery Emphasis: Ensure adequate rest between sessions and prioritize recovery techniques (e.g., foam rolling, stretching) to support muscle repair and growth.

Adjusting your fitness and nutrition plan is essential for overcoming plateaus, maintaining progress, and achieving long-term success in your body transformation journey.

By recognizing signs of stagnation, tweaking nutrition strategies, and modifying workouts effectively, you can optimize your efforts, break through barriers, and continue advancing towards your health and fitness goals. Consistency, adaptation, and commitment to personalizing your plan are key to navigating challenges and achieving sustainable results over time.

Chapter 5: The 12-Week Transformation Program

The 12-Week Transformation Program is designed to guide you through a structured journey of fitness and health improvements. This section focuses on the initial phase, Weeks 1-4, where the emphasis is on building a solid foundation through effective workout plans, nutritional guidelines, meal plans, and tips for staying motivated.

Weeks 1-4: Building a Foundation

Purpose:

- Establish a consistent exercise routine to build strength, improve endurance, and lay the groundwork for progression.

Week 1:

- **Day 1 (Strength Training):** Full-body workout focusing on basic exercises (e.g., squats, push-ups, rows).

- **Day 2 (Cardio):** 20 minutes of moderate-intensity cardio (e.g., brisk walking or cycling).

- **Day 3 (Active Recovery):** Yoga or gentle stretching to promote flexibility and recovery.

- **Day 4 (Strength Training):** Upper body workout with emphasis on chest and arms.

- **Day 5 (Cardio):** HIIT session (e.g., 30 seconds of sprinting followed by 1 minute of walking).

- **Day 6 (Rest or Light Activity):** Active rest day with light walking or recreational activity.

- **Day 7 (Rest):** Complete rest day to allow for full recovery.

Week 2-4:

- Gradually increase intensity, weights, or duration of workouts based on comfort and progression.

- Continue alternating strength training, cardio, and active recovery days to balance muscle development and cardiovascular fitness.

Nutritional Guidelines and Meal Plans

Purpose:

- Support your workout regimen with balanced nutrition to fuel workouts, promote muscle recovery, and achieve optimal health.

Nutritional Guidelines:

- Caloric Intake: Calculate daily caloric needs based on goals (e.g., weight loss, maintenance, muscle gain).

- Macronutrient Balance: Ensure adequate protein intake for muscle repair, balanced with carbohydrates and healthy fats for energy.

- Hydration: Drink sufficient water throughout the day to maintain hydration levels.

Sample Meal Plan (Day):

- **Breakfast:** Whole grain oats with berries and Greek yogurt.

- **Mid-Morning Snack:** Apple slices with almond butter.

- **Lunch:** Grilled chicken breast with quinoa and steamed

vegetables.

- **Afternoon Snack:** Protein shake or Greek yogurt with mixed nuts.

- **Dinner:** Baked salmon with sweet potato and mixed greens.

- **Evening Snack (Optional):** Cottage cheese with fruit.

Tips for Staying Motivated

- **Set Clear Goals:** Define specific, achievable goals for each week and the overall 12-week program.

- **Track Progress:** Use a journal or app to monitor workouts, nutrition, and achievements.

- **Find Support:** Join a fitness community, enlist a workout buddy, or seek guidance from a coach or trainer.

- **Reward Progress:** Celebrate milestones with non-food rewards to reinforce positive habits and motivation.

- **Stay Flexible:** Adapt workouts and meal plans as needed to fit your schedule and preferences.

The first phase of the 12-Week Transformation Program lays the foundation for sustainable progress by integrating structured workouts, balanced nutrition, and motivation strategies.

By following the detailed week-by-week workout plan, adhering to nutritional guidelines and meal plans, and implementing tips for staying motivated, you can establish healthy habits and set the stage for continued success in your fitness journey.

Consistency, dedication, and a positive mindset will propel you towards achieving your desired transformation goals over the course of the program.

Weeks 5-8: Increasing Intensity

Weeks 5-8 of the 12-Week Transformation Program focus on increasing the intensity of both workouts and nutrition strategies to accelerate progress and overcome plateaus. This phase emphasizes pushing your physical limits, refining your nutritional approach, and developing mental resilience to sustain motivation and effort.

Adjusting Workouts for More Intensity

Purpose:

- Enhance strength, endurance, and overall fitness by progressively challenging your body with more intense workouts.

Strategies:

- Increase Weight: Gradually lift heavier weights in strength training exercises to promote muscle growth and strength.

- Higher Reps and Sets: Add more repetitions and sets to your routines to increase volume and workload.

- Advanced Exercises: Incorporate more complex movements (e.g., deadlifts, pull-ups, plyometrics) to target multiple muscle groups.

- Shorter Rest Periods: Reduce rest intervals between sets to maintain elevated heart rate and improve cardiovascular endurance.

Sample Week 5-8 Workout Plan:

- **Day 1 (Strength Training):** Full-body workout with

increased weights and additional sets (e.g., squats, bench press, deadlifts).

- **Day 2 (Cardio):** 30 minutes of high-intensity cardio (e.g., running, spinning).

- **Day 3 (Strength Training):** Upper body with advanced exercises (e.g., pull-ups, shoulder press).

- **Day 4 (Active Recovery):** Yoga or mobility-focused stretching.

- **Day 5 (HIIT):** 20-30 minutes of HIIT (e.g., circuit training with minimal rest).

- **Day 6 (Strength Training):** Lower body with focus on increased intensity (e.g., lunges, leg press).

- **Day 7 (Rest or Light Activity):** Complete rest or light activities like walking.

Advanced Nutrition Strategies

Purpose:

- Fine-tune your diet to support increased training intensity, optimize recovery, and enhance overall performance.

Strategies:

- Macro Adjustments: Increase protein intake to support muscle repair and growth, while adjusting carbs and fats to meet energy demands.

- Nutrient Timing: Focus on nutrient timing around workouts (e.g., carbs and protein pre- and post-workout) to maximize energy and recovery.

- Hydration and Electrolytes: Ensure adequate hydration and replenish electrolytes, especially after intense workouts.

Sample Advanced Meal Plan (Day):

- **Pre-Workout:** Banana with a scoop of protein powder.

- **Breakfast:** Egg white omelette with spinach and whole grain toast.

- **Mid-Morning Snack:** Greek yogurt with chia seeds and honey.

- **Lunch:** Quinoa salad with grilled chicken, avocado, and mixed greens.

- **Afternoon Snack:** Protein smoothie with berries,

spinach, and almond milk.

- **Post-Workout:** Protein shake with a piece of fruit.

- **Dinner:** Grilled fish with roasted vegetables and a side of brown rice.

- **Evening Snack (Optional):** Cottage cheese with sliced cucumber.

Mental Strategies for Pushing Through

Purpose:

- Develop mental resilience and motivation to sustain effort and overcome challenges during intensified training.

Strategies:

- Set Intermediate Goals: Break down your 12-week goal into smaller, manageable milestones to maintain focus and motivation.

- Positive Visualization: Use visualization techniques to mentally rehearse success and overcome mental barriers.

- Mindfulness and Stress Management: Incorporate mindfulness practices, such as meditation or deep breathing, to manage stress and maintain mental clarity.

- Accountability: Continue leveraging support systems, such as workout partners or fitness communities, to stay accountable and motivated.

Increasing intensity during Weeks 5-8 of the 12-Week Transformation Program is crucial for driving progress and overcoming plateaus.

By adjusting workouts for more intensity, implementing advanced nutrition strategies, and developing mental resilience, you can push your limits and achieve significant fitness gains. This phase challenges you to elevate your efforts, refine your approach, and cultivate a strong mindset, setting the stage for continued success in your transformation journey.

Consistency, perseverance, and strategic adjustments will propel you towards your ultimate fitness goals.

Weeks 9-12: Finishing Strong

The final phase of the 12-Week Transformation Program, Weeks 9-12, is all about finishing strong. This period focuses on giving a final push in your workouts, fine-tuning your nutrition for peak performance, and preparing for life after the program. By maximizing your efforts and refining your approach, you can achieve significant results and set the foundation for sustaining your fitness journey long-term.

Final Workout Push

Purpose:

- Intensify your training to maximize strength, endurance, and overall fitness gains as you approach the end of the program.

Strategies:

- Peak Performance Workouts: Increase intensity with maximum effort sessions, pushing your limits in both strength and cardio exercises.

- Supersets and Circuits: Incorporate supersets (two exercises back-to-back without rest) and circuit training to elevate heart rate and enhance muscle endurance.

- Explosive Movements: Add plyometric exercises (e.g., jump squats, burpees) to boost power and agility.

Sample Week 9-12 Workout Plan:

- **Day 1 (Strength Training):** Full-body workout with supersets (e.g., squats followed by lunges, bench press followed by push-ups).

- **Day 2 (Cardio):** 30-40 minutes of HIIT (e.g., sprint intervals, kettlebell swings).

- **Day 3 (Strength Training):** Upper body with added plyometrics (e.g., plyo push-ups, medicine ball throws).

- **Day 4 (Active Recovery):** Dynamic stretching or yoga to maintain flexibility and aid recovery.

- **Day 5 (Strength Training):** Lower body with circuit training (e.g., leg press, step-ups, deadlifts).

- **Day 6 (Cardio):** Long steady-state cardio (e.g., 45-60 minutes of running or cycling).

- **Day 7 (Rest or Light Activity):** Complete rest or light activities like walking.

Fine-Tuning Nutrition for Peak Performance

Purpose:

- Optimize your diet to support high-intensity training, ensure proper recovery, and maintain energy levels.

Strategies:

- Precision Macronutrient Adjustments: Tailor your macronutrient intake to support peak performance, focusing on higher protein for muscle repair, complex carbs for sustained energy, and healthy fats for overall health.

- Micro-Nutrition Focus: Ensure adequate intake of vitamins and minerals to support immune function, muscle function, and overall well-being.

- Hydration Optimization: Maintain optimal hydration, especially before, during, and after intense workouts.

Sample Peak Performance Meal Plan (Day):

- Pre-Workout: Energy bar or a small serving of oatmeal with a banana.

- **Breakfast:** Scrambled eggs with vegetables and whole grain toast.

- **Mid-Morning Snack**: Protein smoothie with spinach, berries, and flaxseeds.

- **Lunch:** Turkey and avocado wrap with a side of mixed greens.

- **Afternoon Snack:** Hummus with carrot and celery sticks.

- **Post-Workout:** Protein shake with a piece of fruit.

- **Dinner:** Grilled chicken with quinoa, roasted vegetables, and a side salad.

- **Evening Snack (Optional):** Greek yogurt with honey and walnuts.

Preparing for Life After the Program

Purpose:

- Transition from the structured 12-week program to a sustainable long-term fitness and nutrition routine.

Strategies:

- Establish Long-Term Goals: Set new fitness and health goals to maintain motivation and continue progress.

- Flexible Routine: Develop a flexible workout and nutrition plan that fits your lifestyle and preferences.

- Sustainability Focus: Emphasize sustainable habits, such as regular physical activity, balanced diet, and mindful eating.

Action Plan:

- Evaluate Progress: Reflect on achievements, challenges, and lessons learned during the 12 weeks.

- Plan Maintenance Workouts: Design a maintenance workout schedule that includes a mix of strength training, cardio, and flexibility exercises.

- Continue Tracking: Keep tracking progress through journals, apps, or wearables to stay accountable.

- Adapt and Evolve: Be open to adapting your routine as your fitness level and goals evolve over time.

The final phase of the 12-Week Transformation Program is about giving your best effort and setting the stage for long-term success.

By intensifying your workouts, fine-tuning your nutrition, and preparing for life after the program, you can achieve remarkable results and establish a sustainable, healthy lifestyle.

Consistency, commitment, and adaptability are key to maintaining the progress you've made and continuing to improve your fitness and well-being beyond the 12-week mark. Finish strong, stay motivated, and embrace the lifelong journey of health and fitness.

Chapter 6: Maintaining Your Transformation

Maintaining your transformation is crucial for preserving the progress you've made and ensuring long-term health and fitness. This section focuses on creating a sustainable lifestyle that integrates fitness and nutrition seamlessly into your daily routine. We'll explore how to transition to a maintenance plan and balance fitness with everyday life, providing you with the tools to sustain your achievements and continue growing.

Transitioning to a Maintenance Plan

Purpose:

- Shift from the intense structure of the 12-week program to a long-term, manageable routine that supports ongoing health and fitness.

Strategies:

- Gradual Adjustment: Slowly reduce the intensity and frequency of workouts while maintaining regular exercise. This helps your body adapt and prevents burnout.

- Balanced Routine: Create a balanced fitness plan that includes strength training, cardio, and flexibility exercises, but with more moderate intensity and volume.

- Consistent Nutrition: Continue to follow a balanced diet, focusing on whole foods and proper portion sizes, but allow for occasional indulgences to maintain flexibility and enjoyment.

Action Plan:

- Weekly Schedule: Plan workouts 3-5 times a week, mixing different types of exercises to keep it varied and enjoyable.

- Monitor Progress: Keep tracking your fitness and nutrition, but with less rigidity. Use apps or journals to maintain accountability.

- Adjust as Needed: Be open to adjusting your plan based on how your body feels and your lifestyle changes. Flexibility is key to sustainability.

Balancing Fitness with Daily Life

Purpose:

- Integrate fitness into your everyday routine without it feeling like a burden, making it a natural part of your lifestyle.

Strategies:

- Time Management: Prioritize workouts by scheduling them at convenient times, whether early in the morning, during lunch breaks, or in the evening. Consistency is more important than the time of day.

- Active Lifestyle: Incorporate physical activity into your daily life. Take the stairs, walk or bike to work, engage in active hobbies, and find opportunities to move throughout the day.

- Family and Social Support: Involve family and friends in your fitness journey. Plan active outings, cook healthy meals together, and support each other's goals.

Action Plan:

- **Daily Routine:** Establish a routine that includes regular physical activity. Even short, 20-30 minute workouts can be effective if done consistently.

- **Meal Prep:** Continue meal prepping to save time and ensure you have healthy options available, even on busy days.

- **Mindful Living:** Practice mindfulness and stress management techniques to maintain mental well-being, which is crucial for overall health and motivation.

Creating a sustainable lifestyle is the key to maintaining your transformation and continuing to thrive. By transitioning to a manageable maintenance plan and balancing fitness with daily life, you can integrate healthy habits seamlessly into your routine.

The focus should be on long-term consistency, flexibility, and enjoyment. Embrace the journey, stay committed to your goals, and enjoy the benefits of a healthier, fitter you for years to come.

Long-Term Goal Setting

After completing a transformative fitness program, setting new long-term goals is crucial to maintaining your progress and continuing to improve. This section will guide you through setting new fitness goals and emphasize the importance of continuing education and staying informed about health and fitness. By setting clear, achievable goals and keeping yourself updated, you can sustain your motivation and adapt to evolving fitness trends and knowledge.

Setting New Fitness Goals

Purpose:

- To keep your fitness journey exciting and challenging by setting new, achievable goals that build on your current progress.

Strategies:

- Reflect on Achievements: Begin by assessing what you've accomplished during your transformation program. Recognize the milestones you've hit and areas where you excelled.

- Identify Areas for Improvement: Determine which

aspects of your fitness or health you'd like to improve further. This could include increasing strength, improving cardiovascular fitness, enhancing flexibility, or achieving specific performance milestones (e.g., running a marathon, lifting a certain weight).

- Set SMART Goals: Use the SMART criteria (Specific, Measurable, Achievable, Relevant, Time-bound) to set clear and structured goals. This approach ensures that your goals are well-defined and realistic.

Action Plan:

- **Specific Goals:** Clearly define what you want to achieve. For example, instead of saying, "I want to get stronger," specify, "I want to increase my bench press by 20 pounds in the next three months."

- **Measurable Progress:** Establish how you will measure your progress. This could be through tracking weights lifted, distances run, body measurements, or other quantifiable metrics.

- **Achievable Targets:** Ensure your goals are challenging yet attainable. Setting unrealistic goals can lead to frustration and burnout.

- **Relevant Objectives:** Align your goals with your overall lifestyle and long-term vision. They should be meaningful and significant to you.

- **Time-Bound Deadlines:** Set a timeframe for achieving each goal. This creates a sense of urgency and helps keep you motivated.

Example Long-Term Goals:

- **Strength:** Increase squat weight by 30 pounds in six months.

- **Endurance:** Run a half-marathon in four months.

- **Flexibility:** Improve hamstring flexibility to touch toes with ease in three months.

Continuing Education and Staying Informed

Purpose:

- To stay motivated, adapt to new information, and continuously improve your fitness and health knowledge.

Strategies:

- Follow Reliable Sources: Keep up with reputable health and fitness websites, blogs, and social media channels. Look for content from certified trainers, nutritionists, and medical professionals.

- Enroll in Courses and Workshops: Participate in online courses, workshops, or seminars that focus on fitness, nutrition, and wellness. This can deepen your understanding and introduce you to new techniques and concepts.

- Read Books and Articles: Invest time in reading books and scientific articles on fitness and nutrition. This helps you stay current with the latest research and trends.

- Join Fitness Communities: Engage with fitness communities, both online and offline. Forums, social media groups, and local clubs can provide support, motivation, and valuable information.

Action Plan:

- **Weekly Learning Schedule:** Dedicate a specific time each week to learning. This could be an hour spent reading articles, watching instructional videos, or attending a webinar.

- **Professional Guidance:** Consider hiring a personal trainer or nutritionist periodically to get personalized advice and stay updated with professional insights.

- **Certifications:** If passionate about fitness, pursue certifications in personal training, nutrition, or specific fitness disciplines (e.g., yoga, pilates).

Example Learning Resources:

- **Websites:** Visit sites like WebMD, Mayo Clinic, and reputable fitness blogs.

- **Books:** Read titles like **"The New Rules of Lifting"** by

Lou Schuler and Alwyn Cosgrove, **"How Not to Die"** by Dr. Michael Greger, or **"The Body Keeps the Score"** by Bessel van der Kolk.

- **Courses:** Platforms like Coursera, Udemy, and NASM offer various health and fitness courses.

Long-term goal setting and continuing education are vital components of maintaining and advancing your fitness journey. By setting new fitness goals, you can keep yourself challenged and motivated.

Staying informed through continuous learning ensures you remain adaptable and knowledgeable about the latest trends and research in health and fitness. Embrace this lifelong journey with enthusiasm and commitment, and enjoy the enduring benefits of a healthy, active lifestyle.

Chapter 7: Building a Healthy Community

One of the most powerful tools in maintaining and enhancing your fitness journey is the support and motivation that comes from a healthy community. Engaging with fitness communities, finding a workout partner or group, and inspiring others with your journey can significantly boost your commitment and enjoyment of a healthy lifestyle. This section will explore how to build and leverage a supportive community to sustain your fitness goals.

Engaging with Fitness Communities

Purpose:

- To connect with like-minded individuals who share similar fitness goals, providing mutual support, motivation, and accountability.

Strategies:

- Join Online Forums and Social Media Groups: Engage

with platforms like Reddit, Facebook, or Instagram, where fitness enthusiasts share tips, experiences, and support. These communities can be a source of inspiration and practical advice.

- Participate in Local Fitness Groups: Look for local running clubs, yoga classes, or gym groups. Being physically present with others can enhance your commitment and make workouts more enjoyable.

- Attend Fitness Events and Workshops: Participate in local or virtual fitness events, workshops, and seminars. These events are great opportunities to learn, connect, and stay motivated.

Action Plan:

- **Identify Interests:** Find communities that match your fitness interests, whether it's weightlifting, running, cycling, or yoga.

- **Active Participation:** Regularly engage in discussions, share your progress, ask questions, and offer support to others. This reciprocity strengthens community bonds.

- **Networking:** Use these communities to network with fitness professionals and enthusiasts who can provide additional guidance and motivation.

Example Communities:

- **Online:** Reddit's **r/fitness**, Facebook groups like **"Fitness Motivation,"** and Instagram hashtags like **#fitfam**.

- **Local:** Running clubs, CrossFit gyms, and community center fitness classes.

Finding a Workout Partner or Group

Purpose:

- To enhance motivation, accountability, and enjoyment by exercising with others.

Strategies:

- Partner with a Friend or Family Member: Exercising with someone you know can make workouts more fun and ensure you both stay committed.

- Join Group Classes: Many gyms and fitness centers offer group classes in activities like spinning, aerobics, or dance. These classes provide a structured environment and group support.

- Use Technology: Apps like Meetup can help you find local workout partners or groups with similar fitness interests.

Action Plan:

- **Set Common Goals:** Align your fitness goals with your partner or group to ensure mutual motivation and support.

- **Schedule Regular Workouts:** Plan and commit to regular workout sessions together. Consistency is key to building a routine.

- **Encourage Each Other:** Celebrate achievements, offer encouragement during challenging times, and hold each other accountable.

Example Activities:

- **Running Buddy:** Meet a friend for regular morning runs.

- **Gym Partner:** Find someone to join you for weightlifting sessions.

- **Group Classes:** Participate in classes like Zumba, spinning, or boot camps.

Inspiring Others with Your Journey

Purpose:

- To motivate and encourage others by sharing your fitness transformation and experiences.

Strategies:

- Share Your Story: Use social media platforms, blogs, or community boards to share your fitness journey, challenges, and successes. Your story can inspire others to start or continue their own fitness journeys.

- Offer Support and Advice: Be open to helping others who seek advice or motivation. Sharing what you've learned can empower others to make positive changes.

- Lead by Example: Demonstrate the benefits of a healthy lifestyle through your actions. When people see your commitment and results, they're more likely to be inspired.

Action Plan:

- **Regular Updates:** Post regular updates on your progress, including photos, workout tips, and motivational quotes.

- **Engage with Followers:** Respond to comments and messages, offering support and encouragement.

- **Host or Participate in Events:** Organize local fitness events or challenges, or participate in community health fairs and fitness expos.

Example Platforms:

- **Social Media:** Instagram, Facebook, TikTok, and personal blogs.

- **Local Community:** Volunteer to lead a fitness class or workshop at a community center.

Building a healthy community is an essential aspect of maintaining and enhancing your fitness journey. Engaging with fitness communities, finding workout partners or groups, and inspiring others with your journey creates a supportive environment that fosters motivation, accountability, and enjoyment.

By connecting with like-minded individuals and sharing your experiences, you can sustain your fitness goals and inspire others to embark on their own paths to health and wellness. Embrace the power of community, and watch your fitness journey flourish.

CONCLUSION

As we reach the end of **"Guide to Total Body Transformation: How to Lose Weight, Build Muscle, and Improve Endurance in Just 12 Weeks for a Fitter and Healthier You,"** I want to take a moment to reflect on the incredible journey we've shared. This book is more than just a guide—it's a pathway to a healthier, more fulfilling life. I am deeply honored to have had the opportunity to guide you through this transformative process.

Throughout these pages, we've delved into the science of weight loss, muscle gain, and endurance, and we've built a strong foundation for sustainable health. We began by assessing your starting point, setting SMART goals, and creating a personalized plan tailored to your unique body type and needs. We explored the vital role of nutrition, the essentials of exercise, and the power of mindset and motivation.

Your journey through the 12-week transformation program has been designed to progressively challenge and empower you, building a solid foundation in the first four weeks, increasing intensity in the middle phase, and finishing strong with a final push. As you transition from the program to a sustainable lifestyle, you are equipped with the knowledge and tools to maintain your progress, set new goals, and continue learning.

We've also emphasized the importance of community—engaging with fitness communities, finding supportive workout partners, and inspiring others with your journey. Building a healthy community around you not only keeps you motivated but also spreads the benefits of a fit and active lifestyle to those around you.

My deepest hope as an author is that this book has provided you with valuable insights, practical strategies, and the inspiration needed to achieve your fitness goals. Your commitment, perseverance, and dedication are commendable, and I am genuinely thrilled to have been part of your transformation.

As you move forward, remember that your health and fitness journey is ongoing. Celebrate your achievements, stay curious, and continue to seek growth. You have the power to create the life you envision, one step at a time.

Lastly, I have a small favor to ask. If you found this book helpful and transformative, please consider leaving a review on Amazon. Your feedback is incredibly valuable and helps others discover the benefits of this guide. Sharing your thoughts and experiences not only supports my work but also inspires others to embark on their own fitness journeys.

Thank you for allowing me to be a part of your journey to a fitter and healthier you. Keep striving for excellence, stay committed to your goals, and enjoy the remarkable benefits of a healthy, active lifestyle!

With gratitude and best wishes,

Maya Harmony